THE CHEMISTRY OF HEALTH

EAT YOUR WAY TO HEALTH AND LONG LIFE

Consider self-healing remedies rather than
medication and side effects

Don Alexander with

Dr. B. D. Alexander

2011

Dedicated to

A public understanding of the chemistry of life.

The information in this book is not intended to replace the advice of health care professionals such as physicians and surgeons.

In some individual health situations, foods described herein may conflict with over the counter and/or prescribed medications.

When in doubt, consult your doctor.

The Chemistry of Health   Don Alexander

TABLE OF CONCERNS

Subject	Page

Introduction & Weight Control

Everything in our universe can be described as either organic (having some form of life) or inorganic (void of any form of life). For example, a rock is inorganic whereas a tree is organic. A wooden railing is inorganic and a fly is organic.

On a more primitive and molecular scale, everything in our universe and on our planet exists either as energy or matter. Energy, on a visible level, can manifest itself as electricity, steam, fossil fuels, etc., and matter can be seen in the form of viruses, bacteria, plants, animals, and humans as well as plasma, gases, liquids and solids.

The truly amazing bit of trivia is that all energy and all matter is composed of microscopic atoms which further break down into subatomic particles which differ only in number of positively charged particles within the nucleus of each atom. The gas, hydrogen, has one such particle while oxygen gas has eight and uranium has ninety-two. The precise number of positively charged atomic particles (named protons) within the nucleus of any atom determines which element (hydrogen, oxygen, lead, gold, silver, iron, sodium, etc. – [total separate elements = 118]) the atom is part of.

The other atomic particles within the atom consist of neutrons (neutral electrical charge) and electrons (negative electrical charge). Neutrons are mixed with protons within the nucleus and electrons orbit or vibrate around the nucleus. The number of neutrons determine whether the element is stable or radioactive and the number of electrons determine which other elements can bond with the specific element being considered. For example, two atoms of hydrogen bonded with one atom of oxygen produce one molecule of water. Molecules of water bonded with molecules of other specific elements (carbon, potassium, iron, zinc, copper, selenium, etc., etc.) make up the human body).

The human body produces billions of human cells (skin, heart, liver, kidney, bladder, blood, lung, etc., etc.) every day as the result of the combining of the basic elements into molecules and compounds (mixture of molecules) which in turn make up individual body cells which make up the whole body (viruses, bacteria, plants, animals, humans, etc.). The basic elements metabolized by the human body into cells are introduced into the body within the food items that humans eat. Therefore, what humans eat determines whether the individual body is strong and healthy or weak and sickly.

Thus, when the human body is deprived of foods containing all the elements required for healthy body cells to multiply and function properly, the body attempts to compensate for the deficiencies by abnormal combining of the elements within the metabolism of processing food into body energy and body matter.

Over the counter and prescription medications consist of the same basic elements that the body and food items consist of; but often in an unhealthy concentrated form which causes minor or major side effects. One side effect of every medication is physical death albeit a very small percentage of individuals ingesting the medication. So, when discussing medications, the benefits are weighed against the inherent risks (a medication with negative side effects may be preferable to a weak and sickly body). On the other hand, natural foods cause few negative side effects other than allergies or bodily imbalance due to overeating (gluttony) or diet deficiencies. Consequently, when eating foods that balance bodily needs is compared against medications, the healing food items win hands down.

The purpose of this book is to provide information on self-healing remedies through food items selection as opposed to ingesting medications and diet supplements which may inflict unwanted side effects. Remember, everything in the universe (which certainly includes both foods and medications) consist of the basic elements such that in many, many instances it is wiser to eat the self-healing foods than to ingest supplements and/or medications.

Juices and extracts from food items also contain the basic elements just like expensive cremes and other compounds that are sold by pharmacies. Therefore, in many instances, there is no particular advantage of pharmacy cremes and compounds over basic food juices and extracts. Oftentimes, doctors prescribe medications over self-healing foods to justify office visit income and because most people do not know or do not consider what the self-healing foods alternatives are. And, of course, there is the placebo effect wherein certain individuals recover from sickness by believing the placebo medication healed the body whereas the sickness was never more than imaginary (hypochondriac).

Choosing self-healing foods over medications can save a lot of money and avoid many unwanted side effects. The best choice of all is to eat healthy every day while at the same time avoiding the temptation to over indulge. Victims of gluttony not only feel quite uncomfortable and self-conscious but also run the risk of serious health problems.

Body weight is directly proportional to calories ingested and the rate of individual metabolism. A high rate tends to retard weight gain and slow metabolism fosters weight gain. There are very few factors that actually affect individual metabolism and food items and/or habitual drugs ingested are more likely to alter individual metabolism than other factors. Diet plays a much bigger role in weight control than exercise.

Consequently, virtually every "diet plan" actually relies on calorie reduction rather than strenuous exercise routines. Exercise without calorie reduction will have a minor effect on weight loss whereas calorie reduction can result in major weight loss without any exercise routine. The fastest way to lose unwanted pounds is to count calories and to eliminate between meals snacks and junk foods which tend to be calorie dense. An exercise routine will help tone body shape and help avoid a flabby appearance from weight loss produced through significant calorie reduction.

An individual who is overweight by a hundred pounds can lose all abnormal body weight within six months through calorie reduction without feeling hungry by following the below menu choices which also provide a healthy and balanced diet. The secret to major weight loss is determination and refusal to "cheat" on menu selections.

For proper nutrition and healthy body, an individual must consume a balanced menu of the basic food groups containing the mixture of chemical elements the body needs for healthy functioning. Fad diets, diet pills and "fat blockers" invariably interfere with healthy metabolism and digestion in addition to robbing the body of essential vitamins, minerals and other essential nutrients while perhaps resulting in minor weight loss that is unnatural and unhealthy.

Weight loss and weight gain is the natural result of total calorie intake over an extended period of time. If you take in more calories than your body needs, you are going to gain weight. Conversely, if you take in fewer calories than your body needs, you are going to lose weight whether you are a jogger or couch potato. Most people know this truism, but what most people do not consider is that the source of the calories does not matter as far as weight gain or loss. It does matter as far as a healthy body is concerned.

To lose weight, all that is necessary is to radically slash calorie intake. The ideal approach is to slash calories, eat a well balanced menu of foods that cover all the basic food groups thus maintaining bodily health, and not to be hungry thereby feeling starved. This can easily be accomplished once the individual is absolutely determined to reduce body weight to a normal level.

Cheating on calorie intake will defeat your calorie reduction plan and you will give up when you experience no weight loss. Another way to become discouraged is to weigh yourself daily. Fluid and feces retention can result in daily weight variation exceeding five pounds. Only weigh yourself naked once a week and do so the first thing when you awaken after urinating and hopefully having a bowel movement.

Your weight will vary during the day. Eating and drinking will increase your body weight because if you consume two pounds of fluids and a pound of food; that combined weight gets on the scale with you; and being fully dressed can add as much as five pounds to your body weight.

The most critical factor of all is your determination to lose unwanted pounds of body weight and to not cheat in any manner until you reach your desired weight. If you do not cheat, the weight will disappear at the rate of five pounds or more each week. Thus, in six months, you can easily lose over 100 pounds. Moreover, you do not actually need to count calories if simply following the menu plan detailed below and do not deviate from it for any reason. Do not eat out. Do not buy or allow in your home any food items that are not on the menu plan. The plan includes all the basic food groups and the specifically selected items on the menu will satisfy your hunger after your stomach shrinks a bit (about three days).

Never, never, never, eat between meals and do not eat after 6:00 pm. Drink fluids with no or very few calories such as black coffee, tea, water, diet soda, or carbonated water. Reduce your salt intake by adding no salt to your food and drink plenty of water, The food on the menu plan has enough salt in it already.

MENU PLAN FOR 900 OR LESS CALORIES DAILY

Breakfast

Option one: Two slices of Best Choice 100% whole wheat toast and two tablespoons of Smucker's sugarless jelly.
Toast – 100 calories; jelly – 25 calories
1/2 cup baby pre-washed carrots, and two stalks of celery.
Carrots – 30 calories; celery – 20 calories
        Total calories – option one = 175

Option two: one cup of Best Choice Rice

Crisps and one cup of 2% milk plus one medium sized orange. Best Choice Rice Crisps – 100 calories; one cup of 2% milk – 100 calories; one medium orange – 60 calories

Total calories – option two = 260

Option three: one cup of blueberries; one cup of cantaloupe pieces; one half grapefruit.
Blueberries – 80 calories; cantaloupe – 60 calories; ½ grapefruit – 40 calories.

Total calories option three = 180

Option four: Two cups of fresh strawberries; one medium tangerine; one cup of blueberries.
Strawberries – 90 calories; blueberries – 80 calories; tangerine – 40 calories.

Total calories option four = 210

Option five: egg sandwich with one egg fried with Pam vegetable spray, two slices of Best Choice 100% whole wheat bread; one cup of fresh strawberries.

Egg – 75 calories; bread – 100 calories; strawberries – 45 calories.

Total calories option five = 220

Breakfast fluids for all options: black coffee, water, tea, or carbonated water.

Lunch

Option one: fresh garden salad with two tablespoons of Wishbone fat free Italian Dressing; one 8 oz. glass of tomato juice;

one cup of fresh strawberries; three stalks of celery. Bagged garden salad, one 9 oz. serving – 60 calories; dressing – 30 calories; strawberries – 45 calories; 8 oz. Glass of tomato juice – 35 calories; three stalks of celery – 20 calories.

Total calories option one = 190

Option two: 1/2 cup baby carrots; four stalks of celery; one banana; one apple. Carrots – 30 calories; celery – 25 calories; one banana –110; apple –75 calories.

Total calories option two = 240

Option three: two boiled eggs; 9 oz. Garden salad; two tablespoons of Wishbone low fat Italian Dressing. Eggs – 150 calories; salad – 60 calories; dressing – 30 calories.

Total calories option three = 240

Option four: 1/2 baby carrots; one cup fresh sliced cucumbers, two cups fresh strawberries; 8 oz. glass of tomato juice; three oz. of radishes. Carrots – 30 calories; cucumber – 15 calories; strawberries – 90 calories; tomato juice – 40 calories; radishes – 25 calories.

Total calories option four = 200

Option five: three oz. tuna packed in water; 9 oz. garden salad; two tablespoons of Wishbone low fat Italian Dressing; two cups sliced cucumbers. Tuna – 100 calories; salad – 60 calories – dressing – 30 calories; cucumbers – 30 calories.

Total calories option five = 220

Fluids with all lunch options: black coffee, water, diet soda with no calories, tea, carbonated water

Dinner

Option one: 6 ounces grilled rib eye steak; ½ cup of asparagus; two cups sliced cucumbers; three ounces of radishes. Steak - 380 calories, asparagus – 20 calories; sliced cucumbers – 30 calories; radishes – 25 calories.

Total calories option one = 455

Combine with breakfast option three and lunch option four.

Total calories for entire day = 840

Option two: 6 ounces of grilled or baked chicken; 4 ounces whole peeled tomatoes; ½ cup of peas; one cup of Green Giant green beans; 3 stalks of celery.

Chicken – 300 calories; tomatoes – 45 calories; green beans – 45 calories; celery – 25 calories; peas – 60 calories.

Total calories option two = 475

Combine with breakfast option three and lunch option one = 845 calories for entire day

Option three: 6 ounces tuna packed in water; 8 ounces of spinach; 8 ounces of cauliflower; 4 ounces peeled whole tomatoes; 3 ounces of radishes. Radishes – 25 calories; tuna – 200 calories; cauliflower – 50 calories; tomatoes – 45 calories;

spinach – 70 calories.

Total calories for option three = 390

Combine with breakfast option two, lunch option three = 900 calories for entire day

Option four: 6 ounces of cured center sliced ham steak; ½ cup asparagus; three stalks of celery; 1/2 cup baby carrots, 4 ounces of cauliflower; Ham – 330 calories; cauliflower – 25 calories; asparagus – 20 calories; carrots – 30 calories; celery – 25 calories;

Total calories option four = 430

Combine with breakfast option one and lunch option one = 795 calories for entire day

Option five: 6 ounces of grilled pork tenderloin; two cups sliced cucumbers, 4 ounces of peeled whole tomatoes; 3 stalks of celery; one cup Green Giant green beans. Tenderloin – 280 calories; cucumbers – 30 calories; tomatoes – 45 calories; green beans – 75 calories; celery – 25 calories.

Total calories option six = 455

Combine with breakfast option five and lunch option five = 895 calories for entire day.

Dinner fluids for all dinner options: diet soda with no calories, water, black coffee, tea, carbonated water.

Stick to this menu and get rid of all your fat while staying healthy and not feeling hungry or discouraged.

When commencing this menu program you must allow about three days for your stomach to shrink before you will be satisfied with food intake and feel comfortable. If you are prone to gain weight, you must carefully control your calorie intake even after you reach your normal body weight. Generally speaking, once your weight goal is achieved, you must limit total calorie intake to around 1,200 calories per day. However, by sticking to the above menu selections plus additional food items selection totaling 300 calories or less your weight should remain stable.

Within the above menu selection you can substitute food items within the same food group (grains, fruits, vegetables, etc.) which contain the same approximate calorie content thereby maintaining your desired weight and eating healthy.

Chapter I

Blood pressure stability and heart health

Normal blood pressure will vary slightly with respect to individuals but should generally be 120 over 80 plus or minus 5 points. The most common factors affecting blood pressure are smoking, obesity, arterial blockage, abnormal fluid retention, lack of bodily exercise, congenital defects, and various forms of heart disease such as arrhythmias, strokes, and general hardening of cardiac arteries. To help maintain healthy heart functions, do not smoke, lose excess body weight, exercise at least 30 minutes each day (walking, treadmill, exercise bike, etc.), reduce sodium intake to 1500 milligrams or less per day, avoid cholesterol rich foods and saturated fat while eating more potassium and calcium rich food items. Add more water-soluble fiber and fish to regular diet, and take aspirin daily (with doctor's approval) to lower the risk of blood clots and adopt mental disciplines that control stress.

Healthy heart food items include olive oil, nuts, garlic, fish, soy foods, red wine, high fiber cereals, prunes, beans, bananas, dates, oranges, cantaloupe, apples, raisins, potatoes, beets, broccoli, spinach, tofu, skim milk, winter squash, oat bran, red, yellow and green vegetables plus dairy products. Minimize intake of fats and red meat in daily diet.

Read food labels to ensure the recommended daily ingestion of essential vitamins and minerals as compared to the label items on a high potency bottle of one-a-day vitamins and minerals at a local pharmacy. Pay special attention to the daily recommended intake of selenium, chromium, magnesium and potassium.

It is very helpful to prepare a "routine shopping list" for weekly diet considerations which can be done during leisure time with easy reference to diet guides and food labels. Such shopping lists help ensure a healthy balance between total calorie intake and essential vitamins and minerals. Remember, your body manufactures living cells every second of every day from the basic elements found within our universe. If you do not get the necessary elements from food intake, the only other options are diet supplements, physicians, surgeons and prescription drugs.

Therefore, avoid all fast food items and carefully read the calories, vitamins and minerals labels on fresh, canned and packaged food items. If this self-discipline is neglected, your food ingestion will be random, unhealthy, and fattening.

Because our physical bodies are manufactured and nurtured by what we eat, the result of a poor diet is unnecessary and expensive medical care to cope with weak and sickly physical states (up to and including premature death).

Weight control concerns – heart health

The quick weight reduction menus listed in the foregoing introduction can be varied on a weekly schedule with substitution of food items from the same food groups. Such substitution items should contain approximately the same calorie content as the original menu items. To avoid feeling hungry after regular meals, eat plenty of high fiber foods such as lettuce, celery, carrots, broccoli, radishes and cucumbers which are very low in calories.

When substituting food items for original

menu items, keep in mind that cheating on total daily calorie intake will result in discouragement, depression, and very minor weight loss. Total daily calories determines weight loss whether the calories come from sugars, fats, proteins or carbohydrates. However, getting maximum daily calories from breads, pastries, and high sugar foods will not provide much bulk and leave you very hungry indeed.

What if your blood pressure is too high now?

Blood pressure that is five to ten points high can often be lowered without medication by eating lots of fruits, vegetables, and whole grains while lowering sodium intake, and reducing saturated fats, sugars, and high cholesterol food items. Blood pressure regulation through food selection can save doctor fees, cost of prescription drugs and unwanted side effects of blood pressure medications (one of the major causes of erectile dysfunction, excessive fatigue, and dizziness). Increasing daily potassium intake can lower blood pressure along with the risks of heart attacks and strokes. High potassium foods include beans, potatoes, avocados, steamed clams, bananas and apricots. For existing blood pressure approximating 140 over 90 or above, blood pressure medication should be resorted to until blood pressure stabilizes around 120 over 80 in the absence of medication.

Omega-3 fatty acids

Eicosapentaenoic acid (EPA) and docosahexaenoic acid (DHA) are polyunsaturated fats that help lower triglycerides which generally rise following meals thereby increasing the risks of heart attack or stroke. Not only do omega-3 fatty acids lower triglycerides, EPA converts to prostaglandins (an anti-inflammatory agent). Omega-3 fatty acids also help prevent arrhythmias, inhibit tumor growth and helps keep cancer cells from spreading.

Fatty fish from cold, deep water contain high levels of omega-3 fatty acids. For example, the total EPA and DHA in grams per half-cup serving for mackerel is 2.5 grams, for herring 1.7 grams, for lake trout 1.6 grams, for chinook salmon 1.4 grams, for lake whitefish and tuna 1.3 grams, for Atlantic salmon and bluefish 1.2 grams. Keep in mind that the actual fat in the above fish, ounce for ounce, compares to the leanest cuts of beef.

Fish oil also has an inhibiting effect on blood clotting but has never been shown to cause uncontrolled bleeding (nor any other health concern). Nevertheless, a doctor should be consulted before beginning routine ingestion of fish oil because some asthmatics have reported an increase in asthma attacks when taking fish oil capsules; and some diabetics have reported elevated blood glucose levels. Fish oil capsules should not be mixed with anticoagulants such as Heparin and Coumadin.

Tomatoes are another food that promotes a healthy heart by reducing the risk of blood clots. Around the seeds within tomatoes is a yellow, jelly-like substance that makes blood less sticky thereby helping to inhibit blood clotting. Replacing saturated fats in the diet with monounsaturated and polyunsaturated fats contained in pecans, almonds and walnuts, along with high levels of fiber, vitamin E, copper and magnesium, lowers LDL cholesterol by ten around percent.

Apples, onions, red wine, teas, grapes and

deeply colored berries contain flavonoids which help to reduce plaque and LDL cholesterol. Whole grains, seafood, and leafy green vegetables help control homocysteine which is an amino acid that damages arterial walls. These vitamin B and B-12 rich foods are also relatively low in calories as compared to other food items containing folic acid.

Two teaspoons of raw honey per day strengthens the heart and helps repair cardiac tissue. Hawthorne berries helps normalize blood pressure, helps repair heart valve defects, inhibits atherosclerosis and strengthens heart muscle. Flaxseed oil and garlic help thin the blood and lessen the risk of blood clots.

A couple of glasses of red wine and sips of champagne per day helps strengthen the heart and regulate cardiac rhythm.

Generally speaking, vitamins and mineral

supplements are a waste of money in the presence of a balanced diet covering all the essential food groups required to maintain a healthy body. However, the labels on high potency one-a-day vitamins are a quick and reliable reference for checking the daily recommended ingestion of both vitamins and minerals. Such handy information helps with menu planning and intelligent grocery shopping.

Substituting diet supplements (vitamins, minerals, etc.) for a balanced diet is unwise because such substitution encourages the consumption of junk foods that are high in calories and low in nutritional value. Consumption of junk food and food items high in sugar and other carbohydrates promotes obesity, heart disease, diabetes, and other serious health problems

Heart healthy foods promote bodily health

in general and can form the foundation for a wonderfully balanced diet. Daily exercise such as walking, jogging, bike riding, treadmill workout, and aerobics are easy to perform and help reduce the risk of heart disease as well as a host of other bodily malfunctions.

Chapter II

Body odor, bad breath, flatulence and heartburn

Controlling natural body odors will be quite difficult in the absence of a daily shower and scrubbing with a good bacterial soap. Individuals that ooze a strong body odor may have to shower twice per day (morning and evening). Deodorants are inadequate to make a dirty individual smell fresh and tend to clog up sweat glands and skin pores.

Contrary to popular belief, it is not sweat that smells but rather the waste products from bacteria living on human skin and eating the traces of carbohydrates, proteins and lipids exuded with body perspiration. Offensive body odor can also be caused by a chemical imbalance resulting from poor diet or from disease causing such chemical imbalance. It is also advisable to use washrags and towels only once before laundering them because they become filled with skin cells and bacterial waste that cause body odor.

Persistent and troubling body odor can be relieved somewhat by tradeoffs in daily diet. Red meats may add to stubborn body odor and raw onions or garlic leave behind a strong and offensive mouth odor. Beverages containing caffeine cause excessive perspiration. Other foods contributing heavily to body odor include fried foods, fatty foods, refined sugars, highly processed foods and foods high in chlorine such as fish, eggs, liver, and beans. Other offensive body odors are associated with tobacco and alcohol.

Foods that do not contribute to body odor are those high in chlorophyll (a natural purifier and odor eliminator) such as parsley, kale, leafy green vegetables, spinach, breads and nuts. In extended social situations it is sometimes necessary to choose between favorite foods, nutrition, weight control and aggravated body odor or resorting to effective deodorants which clog sweat gland and skin pores to inhibit bodily perspiration.

Cleansing of sweat glands and pores by heavy exercise, sauna, or extended hot bath prior to showering will also help control body odor. Flushing bodily systems by drinking lots of water will retard body odor. Shaving body hair will reduce bacterial growth and increase the effectiveness of odor control options.

Some natural deodorants

Plain apple cider vinegar has a lower pH level that kills odor causing bacteria. Dampen a cloth with apple cider vinegar and use the cloth to massage armpits and around other sweat glands. This not only kills odor causing bacteria but also wards off other types of bacteria.

Potassium sulfate crystals massaged under armpits and around sweat glands will also kill odor causing bacteria and absorb perspiration moisture.

Rub armpits and other sweat glands with a slice of lemon or lime to kill odor causing bacteria (smells better than vinegar).

Make a paste from baking soda and water and massage under arms and around genitals. Allow the paste to work for a few minutes, then rinse away with a fresh wet washcloth.

Rub witch hazel or rubbing alcohol (both antiseptic) or Tea tree oil (antimicrobial) or green tea extract under arms and around other sweat glands to kill odor causing bacteria but remember such remedies will not prevent sweating-----just reduce offensive perspiration odor.

An almost infinite variety of perspiration absorbing body powders applied after a fresh shower will reduce body odor but may show through clothing and are not advisable if expecting intimate sexual activity.

Flatulence

The most common causes of flatulence (passing gas through the rectum) are: eating or drinking so rapidly that air is taken into the stomach; eating certain foods that produce carbon dioxide, hydrogen, and methane during digestion; pregnancy, and gastrointestinal disorders including cancer and tumors; other types of bowel obstruction; food allergies; inflammation of stomach lining; hiatal hernia; pancreatic disorders; peptic ulcer; gall bladder disease; and digestive disharmony between small and large intestines including the passage of undigested food from the small to large intestine.

Flatulence not due to a physical condition needing medical treatment can be avoided by not taking air into the stomach and avoiding foods that cause digestive disharmony between the small and large intestines. Foods contributing to flatulence are fiber (especially water soluble), starchy foods (like bread and rice), fruits, artificial sweeteners, brussel sprouts, broccoli, cabbage, beans and foods with high sugar content.

There are natural remedies for flatulence

using spices, oils, brandy and rock salt that substitute for expensive gas relief medications:

mix one teaspoon of dry ginger powder with a pinch of asafoetida and pinch of rock salt in a cup of warm water and drink after meal;

or, two teaspoons of brandy in cup of warm water before going to bed;

or chew fresh ginger soaked in lime juice after meal;

or chew peppermint after meal;

or dry grind a supply of one teaspoon pepper, teaspoon of dry ginger, and teaspoon of green cardamom seeds, then take one half teaspoon of this ground mixture with a cup of warm water one hour after meal.

For abdominal discomfort, blend caraway oil with equal part of peppermint oil and drink one quarter cup.

<u>Bad breath</u>

Because stomach odors can readily pass into the mouth, the same factors causing flatulence can result in bad breath and can be treated with the same remedies. However, other causes of bad breath are more difficult to control such as bad teeth, infected gums, food residue packed between teeth; odor producing bacteria imbedded in tongue, postnasal drip from a cold or allergy, mouth dryness, use of antihistamines, dieting, reduced saliva flow, and sulfur containing foods such as garlic, onions, broccoli, and cabbage.

There are other causes of bad breath (such as tobacco and alcohol) but the above factors are the most common.

The tongue surface is rough and pitted allowing infectious bacteria, viruses, fungi, yeast, food particles, and cellular debris to collect and

cause bad breath as well as gum disease, tooth decay, colds and sore throats. Proper flossing and brushing of teeth, and
rinsing of mouth after meals will reduce problems associated with fungi, yeast, bacteria, food particles and cellular debris but may not eliminate bad breath caused by a tongue load of such odor causing residue.

Tongue cleaning can be accomplished by a plastic teaspoon with the bowl pointing down. Firmly scrape the tongue from back of tongue forward several times and clean spoon with 3.0% hydrogen peroxide between scraping cycles. Rinse with antiseptic fluid followed by a breath mint or chewing gum to promote saliva flow.

Natural breath fresheners include anise seeds, parsley leaves, and cloves. Another breath freshener is brushing teeth with baking soda mixed with ground cinnamon. Make your own mouthwash and breath freshener by mixing equal parts of pure essential oils of peppermint, spearmint, star anise, and pure lemon juice in a small bottle. Shake vigorously, then add three drops of the mixture into a glass of water. Gargle and rinse mouth completely.

Get tooth decay and gum disease treated by dentist.

Chapter III

Cancer prevention

Because the precise cause of various types of cancer remains unknown, the routine treatment for cancer patients as administered by traditional physicians specializing in cancer treatment continues to be radiation treatments and/or surgical intervention. Cancer research, cancer treatments and cancer drugs are big, big business around the globe and there is little economic incentive to prevent cancer through healthy diet or to treat cancer with natural food remedies. Neither is the FDA likely to sanction non-traditional cancer treatment.

The Chemistry of Health   Don Alexander

Cancer is a mysterious biological puzzle and thus there is not a generalized agreement within the medical community as to cause and effect relationship which also means that there may be unknown but effective approaches to not only cancer prevention but cancer treatment also.

Dr. Robert Atkins, inventor of the highly-popular Atkins Diet, stated: "There's a war going on ... The War Against Quackery is a carefully orchestrated, heavily endowed campaign sponsored by extremists holding positions of power in the orthodox hierarchy..... The multimillion dollar campaign against quackery was never meant to root out incompetent doctors; it was, and is, designed specifically to destroy alternative medicine... The millions were raised and spent because orthodox medicine sees alternative,drugless medicine as a real threat to its economic power. And right they are...the majority of the drug houses will not survive." (if people were aware of the natural foods remedies)

And alternative cancer physician, Kurt W. Donsbach, D.C., N.D., Ph.D. says: "Alternative medical therapy has been cast into a position of 'the last resort.' Therefore, an alternative practitioner who gets even a small percentage of his patients well should be looked at with considerable respect, because he has helped those for whom no more could be done by allopathic medicine. In fact, quite the opposite is true. Medical doctors, by and large, classify alternative practitioners as 'quacks,' which is defined by Webster as 'fraudulent doctors.' If a patient goes to an allopathic doctor for months or years and eventually is told, 'there is no more medicine can do for you,' and then that patient turns to an alternative practitioner who helps them and may even cure them - who is the quack? Is it the doctor who treated for months or years at considerable cost and the patient continuously proceeds to a more serious state - or the healer who used "unproven" therapies to achieve results? "

"It is estimated that if people had a choice, lack of demand would shrink Doctors and Drugs to less than 10% of its current size, with the remainder almost entirely related to trauma medicine. That would be a $900,000,000,000.00 (nine hundred BILLION dollar) loss to them. They are not going to take this loss without a good fight."---Dr Richard Shulze, N.D.

Blood serum pH remains relatively constant but body tissue pH will fluctuate with changes in diet. Most cancer patients tested reflected a body tissue pH between 4.0 and 5.0 which is well above the normal range.

Logically, then, it would follow that a diet intentionally low in acidity would not favor cancerous cells. It is not a moronic leap in logic to further predict that a carefully selected low acidity and balanced diet should help prevent cancer cells from forming within oxygen rich body tissues.

Another important consideration is that attempts to prevent and treat cancerous cells with diet control is not likely to be harmful since such an approach relies on a well balanced and healthy diet which avoids meats, dairy products and food items containing high sugar levels.

Antitoxins within certain food items protect body cells from damage caused by unstable molecules called "free radicals" which may lead to cancer. Specific antitoxins modify the molecular structure of free radicals thereby stabilizing them. Some examples of antitoxins are glutathione, lipoic acid, catalase, superoxide dismutase, melatonin, beta-carotene, lycopene, and vitamins A, C, and E.

Cancer cells have an anaerobic, fermentative metabolism and require sugar rather than oxygen to survive. Thus, cancer treatment should be aimed at getting more oxygen into the body tissues harboring cancerous cells. The fundamental causes of cancer involve the substitution of the respiration of oxygen in normal body cells with fermentation of sugar.

No cancer cells exist in which the normal respiration of oxygen is intact. Therefore, cancer can be avoided by maintaining normal respiration of oxygen within body tissues. Since alkaline tissues apparently hold 20 times more oxygen than acid tissues, cancer patients' tissues test out to be more acidic compared to non-cancerous tissues.

Consequently, effective cancer prevention and treatment must result in re-establishing oxygen uptake of infected cells. The challenge is how to accomplish normal respiration of oxygen within body tissues harboring cancerous cells. This does not appear to be overly difficult but can be accomplished by removal of toxins and metals, restoration of missing nutritional elements and raising of oxygen levels.

The blood of seriously ill cancer victims generally lacks phosphatides and lipoproteins whereas blood from a healthy person always contains adequate levels of these essential molecules. The blood of some weak and anemic cancer victims has been observed to contain an abnormal greenish-yellow substance rather than the healthy red hemoglobin that carries oxygen to body cells. When normal levels of phosphatides and lipoproteins were restored by diet adjustment including organic flax seed oil with cottage cheese (must be eaten at same time), tumors began shrinking and weakness with anemia faded in a few months.

Essential fatty acids such as linoleic and linolnic are made harmful to healthy bodily functions by manufacturers in order to extend the shelf life of commercial dietary fats found in margarine, hard shortening, and vegetable oils. Chemical processing of these fats destroys the electron cloud thereby keeping the fats from bonding with oxygen and converting healthy fats to "pseudo fats" which are harmful to healthy tissue. The heart, for example, rejects such fats which then wind up as fatty inorganic deposits on the heart muscle itself.

According to Dr. Johanna Budwig (cancer specialist), "chemically processed fats are not water soluble when bound to proteins. They end up blocking circulation, damaging heart action, inhibiting cell renewal, and impeding the free flow of blood and lymph fluids. The bio-electrical action is these areas slows down and may become completely paralyzed. The entire organism shows a measurable loss of electrical energy which is replenished only by adding active lipids to the diet."

Dr. Bugwig further reasons: "These nutritional fats are vital (lipids). Science has proven that fats play an important role in the normal functioning of the entire body. Lipids are vital for all growth processing, renewal of cells, brain and nerve functions, and even for the sensory organs (eyes and ears), and for the body's adjustment to heat, cold, and quick temperature changes. Our energy resources are based on lipid metabolism. To function efficiently, cells require true polyunsaturated, live electron-rich lipids which are present in abundance ir raw flax seed oil. True polyunsaturated fats greedily absorb proteins and oxygen and pump them through the the system. Lipids are only water soluble and free flowing when bound to protein" (thus the importance of protein-rich cottage cheese in the following recommended cancer prevention and treatment diet).

Dr. Budwig sums up the importance of quality lipids: "When high quality, electron-rich fats are combined with proteins, the electrons are protected until the body requires energy. This energy source is then fully and immediately available to the body on demand, as nature intended."

Dr. Budwig published the following cancer treatment diet that has been hailed as miraculous. Notwithstanding, this diet is not recommended to replace the advice of any attending cancer physician.

General Rules:

The patient has no nourishment on day # 1 other than 250 ml (8.5 ounces) of flax oil with honey plus freshly squeezed fruit juices (no sugar added). In the case of a very ill person, champagne may be added on the first day in place of the fruit juices and must be taken with the flax oil and honey. Champagne is easily absorbable and has a serious purpose here. Sugar is absolutely forbidden. Grape juice may be added to sweeten any other freshly squeezed juices.

Other forbidden food items are: all animal fats, all salad oils, commercial mayonnaise, all meats (chemicals and hormones), butter, margarine, and preserved meats (the preservatives block metabolism of even flax oil).

Freshly squeezed vegetable juices are fine (carrot, celery, apple and red beet). Three times daily, warm peppermint, rose, hips, or grape tea (all sweetened only with honey) is essential; one cup of black tea before noon is fine.

Daily plan:

Before breakfast – a glass of Acidophilus milk or sauerkraut juice is taken. For breakfast – Muesli (regular cereal) overlaid with two tablespoons (30 ml) of flax oil and honey plus fresh fruit according to season (berries, cherries, apricots, peaches, grated apple). Vary the flavo teas as desired or black tea. Add a four ounce (120g) serving of "The Spread' (see recipe below) which may be eaten like a custard or added to other food.   At mid-morning (10:00am), drink a glass of fresh juice (apple, celery, or beet-apple).

Lunch:

Raw salad with yoghurt-Flax Oil mayonnaise (see recipe below). Prepare salad with 'salad greens,' grated turnips, kohlrabi, radishes, and sauerkraut or cauliflower. A fine powder of horseradish, chives, or parsley may be added for flavor.

Cooked meal course (lunch):

Steamed vegetables, potatoes, or grains such as rice, buckwheat, or millet to which is added "The Spread" (see below) or the Mayo (see below) for flavor and to up the intake of flax oil. For a hearty meal, mix 'The Spread' with potatoes and add caraway, chives, parsley, or other herbs.

For dessert, mix fresh fruit (other than those eaten at breakfast) with 'The Spread' but instead of using honey flavor with cream of lemon, vanilla or berries.

Afternoon tea --- (early afternoon – 4:00pm): Drink small glass of natural wine (no preservatives) or champagne or fresh fruit juice with one to two tablespoons of honey-coated flax seeds.

Dinner (around 6:00 pm):

Make a hot meal using buckwheat, oat or soy cakes. Grits from buckwheat are the very best and be placed in vegetable soup or in a more solid form of cakes with herbal sauce. Sweet sauces and soups can always be given for more healing energy by adding 'The Spread.'   Only honey or grape juice can be used for sweeteners. No sugar (either brown or white) may be used. Only freshly squeezed juices may be used (never reconstituted juices because of preservative danger). All juices must be completely natural.

How to prepare 'The Spread':

Place 250ml (8.5 oz) flax seed oil into a mixing bowl and add one pound (450 g) of 1.0% cottage cheese (low fat) and four tablespoons (60 ml) of honey. Start mixer and add just enough low fat milk or water to get the contents of the bowl to blend together. Let sit five minutes and taste the oil (should be no oily ring around rim of bowl). Alternatively, yoghurt may be substituted for cottage cheese in proportions of one ounce (30 g) of yoghurt to one tablespoon (15 ml) of flax seed oil and one tablespoon of honey blended per above instructions. Note: when flax seed oil is blended like this, it does not cause diarrhea even when given in large amounts. It reacts chemically with the proteins of the cottage cheese, yoghurt, etc.

How to prepare 'The Mayo':

Mix together two tablespoons (30ml) flax seed oil, two tablespoons milk, and two tablespoons yoghurt. Add (2.5 g) mustard plus some herbs such as marjoram or dill. Then add two or three slices of health food store pickles (absolutely no preservatives --- read label!!) plus a pinch of herbal salts.

The above diet must be maintained for five years or so at which time the tumor(s) may have disappeared. Persons who break the rules of this cancer treatment diet   (eating candy, preserved meats, etc.) will sometimes grow rapidly worse and cannot be saved after they come back from their spree (according to Dr. Budwig).

The above diet is aimed at cancer treatment. However, simple logic dictates that avoiding the foods banned in the treatment diet should also prevent cancers from forming. Daily consumption of flax seed oil eaten with cottage cheese should be a tasty cancer inhibitor due to the positive   impact on normal oxygen respiration within body tissues.

Moreover, though the treatment diet may become monotonous over the five year recommended period, simple cancer prevention is not so stringent. All that should be necessary is avoiding all the food items banned in the treatment diet (especially all types of preservatives) and eating a healthy menu consisting of fresh fruits and vegetables (including freshly squeezed juices), honey for sweeteners, whole grains, nuts, fresh sea foods (heavy on deep water fish), plenty of flax seed oil mixed with cottage cheese, tasty salads with herbal seasonings, teas recommended in cancer treatment diet, yoghurt and desserts low in fats and sugars. What is not eaten? ---- all kinds of animal meats and fats (except fresh seafood), all types of preservatives, raw sugars, commercially altered oils, butters, margarine, hard shortenings, mayonnaise, and whole milk (with butterfat).

Chapter IV

Colds and influenza:

The major discomforts associated with chest, nose and throat are due primarily to cold and flu viruses. The best protection against influenza is a flu vaccine that is effective against known circulating flu viruses or a vaccine developed especially for newly discovered viruses.

Antibiotics that combat bacterial infections are not effective against the more than two hundred cold-causing viruses. Most of the over-the-counter medications as well as prescription medications merely relieve to a limited extent the bodily discomforts common to colds and influenza. The "suffering cycle" for virus infections usually last four to seven days during which the body's natural immune system fights off the infection.

Viruses are actually "encapsulated proteins" that lack internal DNA but utilize the virus' RNA after invading host cells to replicate the virus by "messenger RNA" direction of host cell DNA. The body's immune system recognizes and attacks the foreign proteins.

Consequently, one of the best approaches to combating colds and influenza is to load up on immunity boosting foods like yoghurt containing lactobacillus reuteri, acerola (small cherry like fruit loaded with vitamin C), fresh orange juice, red wine, hot chicken soup, and chamomile tea. Hot chicken soup tends to keep white blood cells from causing inflammation and congestion in the airways. Red wine is credited with stopping influenza cells from replicating.

Chewing honeycomb helps relieve breathing tract stuffiness and provide immunity to allergy producing germs (honeycomb is most effective when it comes from local hives).

Frequent doses of honey stirred into hot lemon juice helps relieve nagging cough. Relieve a sore throat and/or sinus drainage with one teaspoon of vinegar in a glass of water and use as an hourly gargle.

For bad chest cold or flu, mix a healing soup consisting of four garlic cloves and two medium onions in two quarts of water and boil for one hour. Then add a handful of rice and cook until very tender. Ingest in small amounts until fever breaks.

The Chemistry of Health   Don Alexander

To relieve chest wheezing, boil the stems of sweet cherries for two minutes then strain and sweeten the liquid with honey. Take by teaspoons to relieve the wheezing.

For sore throat treatment, mash a clove of garlic into a half cup of honey. Stir in the juice from one fresh lemon and take by teaspoonfuls to sooth pain and inflammation.

Drink tea made from slippery elm bark to fight aches and fever brought on by influenza.

Boil flowers of the marigold plant and then strain. Stir in a tablespoon of honey and a teaspoon of vinegar. A couple of spoonfuls every half hour will moderate a light fever.

Toast thinly sliced bread and butter on both sides. Cover with scalded milk and spoon feed to an individual suffering with flu fever and aches.

The Chemistry of Health   Don Alexander

Hot chicken soup contains an amino acid similar to acetylcysteine (a drug that thins mucus and clears lungs). The soup helps release fluids within the body which drain chest of fluid and retard the formation of mucus.

Warm onion soup (one onion minced with honey on low heat for 40 minutes) is an excellent cough syrup taken one spoonful at a time until cough clears up. Onions are loaded with expectorate and antimicrobial properties which, when ingested warm, increases blood flow to chest and throat.

Osha root stimulates the circulatory system while increasing perspiration, relieving chills, and thinning mucus in lungs and sinuses plus soothing sore tissues. A spoonful three times per day chases coughs, sore throats, congestion and other cold symptoms.

Brew fresh or dried thyme leaves into a tea and sip during the entire day to relieve a chronic cough. Another cough remedy can be made from anise or aniseed. In tea form it adds an anesthetic quality to the remedy. However, chronic use of the remedy can be toxic and ingestion should be limited to one week.

Combine equal parts of honey with wild cherry bark syrup. Then mix in two grams of apricot seed, an ounce of garlic tincture, and ounce of osha root tincture. Store in airtight container and take two spoonfuls every few hours during prolonged coughing spell.

For a natural antibiotic, mix 60 drops of white sage tincture into cup of warm water and drink as a tea or gargle vigorously.

The rinds of citrus fruits contain essential

The Chemistry of Health   Don Alexander

oils, bioflavonoids and vitamin C which can naturally clear up stuffy sinuses and respiratory tracts. Grind or grate the peelings and add a teaspoon to a cup of herbal tea or combine with wild cherry bark syrup for a fruity tasting cough formula.

Oregano can also relieve a cough. Mix a teaspoon of dried oregano into a cup of hot water and steep into a tea. Strain before sipping. Consume up to three cups a day during a cold or coughing spell.

Tea made from ground apricot seeds will suppress a dry, hacking cough. A third of one gram of ground seeds steeped in a cup of hot water is sufficient. Buy the ground seeds at a health food store or buy fresh apricots and grind the seeds in a sturdy blender.

Isatis root tincture contains natural antibacterial and antiviral properties for relieving respiratory rattles caused by a respiratory infection. Take 35 drops every few hours for severe bronchial infection. The root is very bitter and is best taken by dropping the tincture onto the tongue followed by an immediate glass of juice to chase the bitterness.

To formulate a natural medicinal vapor to help clear congestion and bronchial coughs, place a few drops of essential oils like eucalyptus or thyme into a bowl of hot water and breathe for ten minutes or so. Both eucalyptus and thyme contain antimicrobial qualities that fight an infection.

For a persistent hacking cough that robs you of breath several time a day, place a few drops of essential oil of frankincense on a handkerchief and inhale every hour as needed.

The Chemistry of Health   Don Alexander

A teaspoon of wild cherry bark syrup every few hours provides a sweet treatment from a scratchy throat and persistent cough. However, essence of cherry cough drops with sugar coating will have little effect.

To treat a tickle in the throat, make a tea of slippery elm bark or suck a lozenge made from the bark. The soothing tea or lozenge coats the throat and quiets coughing spells.

Note: All of the above cold and flu remedies should be continued for several days after symptoms disappear. Viral infections can flare up again if the cause of infection is not totally neutralized which usually requires three to seven days.

Chapter V

Hair and scalp care:

During the normal lifetime, an individual's hair on the head grows approximately 25 feet. We lose around 100 scalp hairs each day which normally grow back. Our hair is resistant to most everything except fire but may appear lifeless, unmanageable and unhealthy. Although around 90% of baldness is probably hereditary and a dry, itchy scalp results from a variety of diverse factors, there are a surprising variety of home remedies that are reported to work as good as expensive shampoos, creams and medications.

Dry hair and scalp are generally caused by

constant exposure to sun and wind plus the minerals and chlorine in bath and shower water, hair treatment chemicals (like perms), peroxide bleach, and hair developer or relaxer chemicals.

Remember that every physical state in our universe including our physical bodies, bodily functions, sickness, disease and every other health problem result from what we eat and the chemicals (molecular combining of the elements) we are exposed to wherein there exists an exchange of electrons or fusing of protons and neutrons. This truism dictates that our very existence and our physical health is directly related to chemicals within what we eat and the chemicals to which we interact within our personal environment.

Thus, using hard water for bathing can cause dry hair and scalp due to the chemicals in the water. For example, Hard water contains calcium which causes hair to feel dry and heavy. Calcium can cause a perm to relax. It builds up on the scalp and causes flaking giving the appearance of dandruff. Calcium can choke hair at the follicle causing the hair to break off thereby inhibiting the growth of replacement hair.

Hair replacement and growth cycles can be adversely affected by hormonal changes, scalp inflammation that scars hair follicles, autoimmune disorders, emotional and/or physical shock, stretching hair too much for hairstyling, poor nutrition, medications, chemicals used in hair treatment, persistent scalp infection, and trichotillomania (hair pulling mental disorder) plus various genetically determined factors.

Instead of spending a fortune with "hair restoration" professionals/doctors, the following remedies using natural foods for self-healing are endorsed by numerous individuals.

Mix a "hair growing" elixir by combining a quarter cup of onion juice with one tablespoon of honey. Massage daily into scalp, cover head and let elixer work overnight, then wash hair with gentle shampoo and soft water.

For a Russian praised "hair growing" treatment, mix one tablespoon of honey with one jigger of vodka and the juice from a medium-size onion. Massage into scalp every night; cover, sleep, awaken, shampoo and rinse.

An Asian treatment to reduce hair loss is rubbing sesame oil into scalp nightly and covering head with a towel. Wash in the morning with a herbal shampoo and rinse with one tablespoon of apple cider vinegar in one quart of warm water.

An optional recommendation is equal

amounts of olive oil and oil of rosemary shaken vigorously and massaged into scalp. Cover head, sleep, awaken, shampoo and rinse.   Another version substitutes garlic oil obtained from a couple of garlic pearls for the olive oil and oil of rosemary. Another version substitutes one jigger of vodka mixed with a half teaspoon of cayenne pepper massaged into scalp. The vodka and pepper stimulates the scalp blood supply which feeds the hair.   A similar approach is rubbing half a raw onion into scalp, covering head and allowing the onion to stimulate scalp overnight, then shampoo and rinse in morning.

For dandruff treatment:

Squeeze out juice from one large lemon, apply half to hair and mix other half with two cups of warm water. Wash hair with gentle shampoo and rinse with plain water, then rinse again with the water and lemon juice mixture. Repeat process every other day until dandruff disappears.

Massage four tablespoons of warm corn oil into scalp; wrap warm, wet towel around head and wait half hour, then shampoo and rinse. Repeat treatment once per week until dandruff clears up.

Before going to bed, grate piece of ginger and squeeze it through cheesecloth to collect juice to mix with equal amount of sesame oil. Rub mixture into scalp and cover head with cap or towel; sleep, awake, wash hair with herbal shampoo and rinse; then rinse again with one tablespoon of apple cider vinegar mixed with one quart of warm water. Repeat every other day until dandruff vanishes.

Prepare chive tea using one tablespoon of fresh chives with one cup of boiled water; cover and let steep for twenty minutes; then strain and rinse through hair following fresh shampoo.

Mix one part potent mouthwash with ten parts of tap water and massage into scalp after shampooing and leave the residue in hair. Relieves itchy scalp and dandruff without leaving hair sticky.

Mash a handful of peppermint leaves into some vodka and steep for one day. Shake well and add water until liquid looks cloudy, massage into scalp after shampoo and leave mix in hair.

Add one tablespoon of dry sage to one cup of boiled water. Steep for a half hour and strain. Add some antibacterial tea tree oil (few drops) and massage into hair. Do not rinse out.

Dry hair:

The Chemistry of Health   Don Alexander

Shampoo and towel-dry hair. Then, massage one tablespoon of mayonnaise evenly through hair and leave on for one hour. Then shampoo and rinse. The flow of oil from the sebaceous glands should increase while the natural fatty acids in mayonnaise nourish hair.

Mix dried spearmint leaves into a cup of boiled water. Steep for half hour and strain. Massage into freshly washed hair and do not rinse.

Dull, permed hair:

Shampoo, rinse and then rinse again with one cup of apple cider vinegar mixed in two cups of water to resurrect dull hair and leave shiny. Works for permed hair or any lifeless looking hair.

Frizzy, dry hair:

Shampoo and then massage scalp with one

tablespoon of wheat germ oil; then rinse with one half cup of apple cider vinegar stirred into two cups of water to eliminate frizzy appearance.

Hair revitalizing treatment:

Warm up a half cup of olive oil and pour into eyedropper bottle, then let stand in near boiling water for ten minutes. Use eyedropper to squeeze warm oil into hair while vigorously massaging into scalp. After entire head is fully oiled, shampoo and rinse.

Miscellaneous recommendations:

Avoid using rubber bands for hair styling because the rubber insulates some hairs causing them to break easily. Do not comb wet hair because the hairs are stretched out and break off.

To remove gum from hair, rub peanut

butter into the gum, then vigorously rub the gum and peanut butter combo between fingers until the gum is well coated and slips out of hair. Then, shampoo and rinse.

Add one tablespoon of baking soda into soaped up hair and then rinse thoroughly to get rid of hair spray buildup.

Rub hair with a sheet of fabric softener to eliminate static electricity causing hair to be frizzy.

To keep gray hair from yellowing, add a couple teaspoons of laundry bluing to a quart of warm water and use as final rinse after shampooing.

To get rid of perm odors, massage tomato juice into hair and scalp, then cover with plastic bag for fifteen minutes. Rinse hair thoroughly and shampoo, then rinse again.

Chapter VI

Kidneys and bladder concerns:

Kidney stones, kidney and bladder infections are quite common and can be treated in most cases with home remedies if addressed before the conditions become acute. Regular ingestion of pure cranberry juice has proven very effective in preventing both kidney stones and urinary tract infections. To appreciate why and how self-healing remedies work, it is helpful to review the physiology of kidneys and bladder.

The kidneys are located about waist level and are separated by the spinal cord. These small organs remove waste and excess water from the blood and eliminate them as urine. Proper kidney functioning is vital to blood pressure regulation and kidneys are sensitive to changes in blood sugar level. Both hypertension and diabetes can interfere with kidney functions and damage the organs. Separate ureter tubes drain urine from kidneys to the bladder which collects and stores urine until bladder pressure triggers urination by contraction of the muscle lining the bladder thereby expelling the urine outside the body through the penis or vagina.

The urethra (a small tube connecting the bladder with the urine ejection site) and the urinary sphincter (a muscle located at the junction of the bladder and urethra) must relax at the same time the bladder contracts to expel urine. Any section of this urinary tract can become infected and the closer to the bladder the infection is the more serious the condition. An infection along the upper urinary track can easily affect the kidneys causing fever, chills, nausea, vomiting and other severe symptoms.

The lower urinary tract contains the bladder and urethra where infection generally is confined to these entities. Lower urinary tract infections are generally less severe and easier to treat than upper tract infections. Simple infections in healthy urinary tracts usually do not spread to other parts of the body whereas upper tract infections can become serious and complicated.

Complicated infections are generally associated with anatomic abnormalities, can spread beyond the urinary tract, are worsened by underlying medical problems, are resistant to some antibiotics and are more difficult to cure. Such infections should be treated by an urologist.

On the other hand, simple infections can be addressed by self-healing remedies that have proven effective. In the U.S. over seven million urinary tract infections are treated by doctors and other health care professionals per year, and are more common to adults than to children. Infections in children are generally more serious and more likely to require the attention of a physician. Such infections rank second only to respiratory disorders as the most common. Roughly 40% of women and 12% of men will experience a urinary tract infection during their lifetime. The higher incidence among women is believed to be associated with a shorter urethra in females.

Kidney stones are associated with diet, age and parental genetics. Such stones consist of a hard accumulation of calcium and other body solids and can be squeezed along the urinary tract causing extreme pain during urination. Kidney stones can also cause back pain, stomach pain, fever and nausea. Blood in the urine (bright red) is indicative of one or more kidney stones. The burr like exterior of the stones can scrape along the tract causing the bleeding.

Food items that are credited with preventing formation of kidney stones are cranberry juice (without preservatives) and parsley when consumed daily. High acid cranberry juice kills infection causing bacteria and parsley inhibits bacterial replication. A considerable number of home remedies for both prevention of and treatment of simple urinary tract infection are being reported as effective:

Steep a handful of corn silk in three cups of boiled water for five minutes. Strain and drink the three sups throughout the day. Corn silk should be stored in a glass jar and not refrigerated. Corn silk extract is available at health food stores if corn silk is not readily available (like in winter). Use 10 tot 15 drops of corn silk extract to each cup of hot water. It is recommended to urinate before and after sexual intercourse.

Take two teaspoons of apple cider vinegar and immediately eat some plain yoghurt plus drink lots of water and cranberry juice twice a day until infection clears up.

Take two teaspoons of oil of oregano with two odorless garlic capsules three times per day to prevent and cure urinary tract infection.

Drink a fifth of wine before going to bed and the infection will be eliminated overnight by the high alcohol content.

Boil equal parts of hibiscus leaves and water in quart pot.. Let steep for fifteen minutes, then strain leaves and drink three cups a day until quart of fluid is consumed.

Drink a glass of cranberry juice twice a day. Mix two tablespoons of apple cider vinegar with one teaspoon of raw honey in eight ounces of warm water. Drink all of the fluid at on time and repeat three times a day.

Stir half a teaspoon of baking soda in eight ounces of water and drink at one time. Repeat every two hours until infection vanishes.

Make a hot tea from fresh lemon juice using eight ounces of water and two tablespoons of lemon juice. Drink this tea three times a day for several days.

Mix one tablespoon of red vinegar and one tablespoon of honey in eight ounces of hot water three time a day. Take small to medium drinks slowly to avoid vomiting.

Sexual satisfaction:

Other than simply lacking natural sex drive, the main reasons for erectile dysfunction among men over fifty are high blood pressure medications, chronic depression, and side effects from miscellaneous prescription drugs as well as some over-the-counter medications. Any chemicals ingested whether alcohol, medications or controlled substances that inhibit the normal blood flow which engorges the spongy tissue causing a penile erection can and most probably will result in erectile dysfunction. As long as such inhibiting chemicals are ingested, erectile dysfunction will continue to a greater or lesser degree.

Factors affecting erectile dysfunction

involving blood pressure and the need for blood pressure medications are best addressed by the natural lowering of blood pressure through weight reduction, exercise and eliminating foods that contribute to buildup of cholesterol which restricts blood flow by clogging veins and arteries.

When lack of sexual fulfillment is due to lack of sex drive, there are a number of dietary recommendations reported to result in more sexual awareness on the part of both sexes, However, there exists a wide difference of opinions as to the effectiveness of food aphrodisiacs above and beyond the "placebo effect." Food aphrodisiacs are believed to trigger the release of chemicals in the brain which stimulate sexual desire. This is quite possible and rational since chemicals derived from foods in the form of atoms, molecules and compounds (which in turn are the result of chemical interaction between the elements) initiate and regulate every bodily function.

Some foods believed to enhance male sexual arousal are:

vegetables containing androstenone such as celery, asparagus, carrots, and cucumbers;

natural corn juice which contains a lutenizing hormone;

kale, radishes, and spinach which have a tonic effect on the adrenal gland which maintains a triangular secretion interaction with the gonads (sex glands) and pituitary gland;

bananas, avocado, pomegranate, figs, papaya, and peach;

nuts such as gingko and pine;

whole grains such as oats;

shellfish like oysters, caviar, and shrimp;

spices such as cardamom, chili, pepper, and asafetida

Women are believed to be sexually aroused to some detectable level by the smell of almonds, eating chocolate, and drinking champagne or red wine.

Logically, the most likely dietary aphrodisiacs are the foods, herbs and spices that increase the secretion of hormones associated with sexual arousal; and those foods (like celery) that lower blood pressure and/or relax arteries.

It is undetermined whether such alleged aphrodisiacs are as effective in increasing sexual awareness as anxiety and depression avoidance and maintaining an optimum blood pressure and/or practicing good interpersonal relations coupled with sensitivity to an intended partner's emotional characteristics.

Chapter VII

Skin care:

There are hundreds of food items, cosmetics, peels, compacts, lotions, creams, powders and miscellaneous prescription drugs for routine skin care and treatment of wrinkles, blemishes, acne, cancers, rashes, psoriasis, and other undesirable skin conditions. This book will only address natural food items that promote smooth, healthy, and attractive skin. These food items contain vitamins A, C, and E, omega-3 fatty acids, iron, zinc and other elements necessary for daily skin cells nutrition.

Strawberries, citrus fruits, red peppers and

broccoli are excellent food items for smooth skin texture and contain vitamin C which is necessary for the formation and production of collagen, the skin's support system.

Squash, sweet potatoes, and spinach are loaded with beta-carotene, an antioxidant which converts to vitamin A and enhances regular cell production and turnover of skin surface.

Almonds, hazelnuts, and sunflower seeds contain vitamin E and antioxidant that protects skin from UV rays that spawn free radicals. Omega-3 fatty acids in fish oils and ground flax seed fight free radicals that cause inflammation which contribute to aging of skin by attacking collagen.

Wild salmon, Atlantic mackerel, and walnuts retard skin wrinkling. Carotenoids in fortified cereals, lean meat, pork, poultry, and oysters help skin maintain a youthful glow. The iron zinc, and other elements in such foods are essential to healthy cell production and natural sloughing of skin to reduce dullness. Red blood cells need iron for hemoglobin which carries life sustaining oxygen to body cells.

Low glycemic menu planning (more whole wheat grains, proteins, fruits and vegetables rather than enriched white bread, refined sugars and carbohydrates) reduce acne. A sample daily menu following the above recommendation would look like this:

Breakfast:

one cup whole grain fortified cereal

The Chemistry of Health   Don Alexander

one cup of skim milk

one cup of sliced strawberries

one cup of green tea

Lunch:

grilled chicken breast with mustard

two slices whole grain bread

half a fresh tomato

half of fresh avocado

3 leafs of lettuce

one medium apple

Dinner:

     5 ounces wild salmon

     spinach salad tossed with one teaspoon olive oil &   balsamic vinegar

     one medium baked sweet potato

     half cup of sliced red bell pepper

     half cup chopped tomato

     half cup broccoli

Snack/dessert

     8 ounces non-fat plain yoghurt

     1 ounce sunflower seeds

one small orange or cup of baby carrots

1 ounce dark chocolate

glass of red wine

Stomach and digestive tract concerns:

Acid indigestion (heartburn) is generally believed to usually follow overeating and/or consumption of spicy hot foods, hot peppers, overly greasy foods, foods with high acidity, and over indulgence of alcoholic beverages. Indigestion can also be caused by excessive fatigue, food allergies, ulcers of the esophagus or stomach, excessive secretion of digestive acid in stomach, and miscellaneous other digestive system disorders.

More than 100 trillion bacteria within the human digestive tract enhance the process of food metabolism. Two extremely beneficial species known as Lactobacillus acidophilus and Bifidobacterium inhibit growth of the fungus Candida albicans and other harmful microbes. They prevent food poisoning by producing natural antibiotics to control salmonella and other pathogens while boosting immune functions in the intestines. They also synthesize vitamins A, B and K essential to healthy skin, vision, blood clotting, bone formation; facilitate absorption of minerals; break down protein into amino acids; create lactic acid from lactose; help regulate bowel functions and help prevent cancer by limiting the growth of bacteria that produce cancer-causing nitrates. They also metabolize and eliminate carcinogens such as pesticides.

Consequently, it is extremely important to make sure beneficial bacteria reproduce faster than they die. This is accomplished by eating lots of fruits, vegetables, and fermented foods such as yoghurt, sauerkraut, tofu, miso (a soy-based condiment), tempeh (soybean cake), tamari (a type of soy sauce), and pickles. Sodium benzoate destroys beneficial bacteria in fermented foods so select brands that contain no preservatives.

Avoid sugar and alcohol because disease-causing bacteria and fungi feed on sugar; and especially refined sugar (like in table sugar, sweets and alcohol). Avoid all foods made with refined flour like white bread and pasta.

Drink lots of green tea which contains polyphenols that help maintain a balance of beneficial bacteria in the gastrointestinal tract. In addition, catechins in green tea help fight off cancer, control blood sugar, and strengthen bones. Drink four cups each day. Green tea may be supplemented by ginseng tea which also promotes friendly bacteria.

Ginger helps strengthen the lower esophageal sphincter muscle which keeps stomach acid from backing up and causing heartburn. Twice a week, eat a half teaspoon of powdered ginger or make a ginger tea using a half teaspoon to one cup of hot water. Let tea steep for ten minutes.

Heartburn medications generally work by blocking production of stomach acid which can also retard absorption of nutrients. Licorice extract (not licorice candy) can sooth the upset stomach by making the digestive tract more resilient.

Baking soda also provides a heartburn quick remedy. Mix one teaspoon in four ounces of water and stir until the baking soda is completely dissolved. Then, drink the glass empty. Do not exceed 8 teaspoons in any 24-hour period.

Another remedy is prepared from two teaspoons of meadowsweet flowers to one cup of boiling water. Steep 10 minutes, drain and sip cup dry.

To make an acid blocker (for especially stubborn heartburn), mix a teaspoon of slippery elm root powder with a teaspoon of honey and ingest the mixture to coat the digestive tract and sooth away the acid indigestion.

Other natural remedies for digestive system upset are:

Treat an upset stomach with rhubarb tea with a half teaspoon of baking soda mixed in.

To treat nausea and vomiting use cup of strong slippery elm bark tea mixed with two tablespoons of honey, a quarter teaspoon cinnamon, and quarter teaspoon of ginger. Take small sips to settle stomach.

Add a teaspoon of spearmint vinegar to 8 ounces of water and drink down to calm stomach and digestive tract.

Use a tablespoon of clove vinegar to stop vomiting attack.

Sip some peppermint or ginger tea as an after dinner drink to sooth stomach cramps.

For acid indigestion, thoroughly chew a teaspoon of dry rolled oats and swallow to quickly neutralize excess stomach acid.

The Japanese radish daikon is an effective

digestive aid when eating deep-fried foods. Take a grated teaspoon full or eat a couple of slices with your meal.

Slowly sip a cup of hot herbal sage tea to relieve upset stomach.

For sour stomach chew some anise seeds, cardamom seeds or caraway seeds. This will also sweeten mouth and breath.

Raw potato juice will neutralize excess stomach acid. Grate a potato and squeeze it through cheesecloth to capture the juice. Mix one tablespoon of potato juice with half a cup of warm water. Drink down slowly.

Eating a large raw radish will soothe indigestion. Follow radish with a cup of chamomile or peppermint tea.

Fresh papaya juice will help combat indigestion because it contains papain which is a potent digestive enzyme.

If you are not a pregnant woman, sip some white wine after a meal to overcome indigestion. Pregnant women and women nursing a baby should not drink any alcohol.

To settle an upset stomach, combine one tablespoon of arrowroot with enough water to make a paste. Boil the mixture, let cool and add one tablespoon of lime juice before swallowing down.

For chronic indigestion, take a couple of odorless garlic capsules after lunch and before dinner. Use garlic in salads and for seasoning various dishes at every opportunity. Pass on this remedy if garlic upsets your stomach.

The Chemistry of Health   Don Alexander

Scrub some orange peel and eat some after a meal to fight indigestion.

Digestion can be smoother by eating some boiled or steamed zucchini sprinkled with raw grated almonds as side dish.

One quarter teaspoon of cayenne pepper added to soup or sprinkled on food aids digestion.

Add fresh basil to food while cooking to make meal more digestible and prevent constipation.

Digestion of raw vegetables is enhanced by sprinkling fresh lemon juice on the veggies three hours before eating.

Take one tablespoon of extra-virgin, cold pressed olive oil fifteen minutes before a spicy meal (like Mexican food) to avoid spicy indigestion.

One teaspoon of whole white mustard seeds taken before a meal may prevent stomach distress resulting from eating foods likely to trigger indigestion.

When eating a spicy meal likely to trigger heartburn, add some turmeric to the food. Turmeric stimulates the flow of saliva which aids digestion and helps balance digestive juices.

To relieve stomach cramps, pour one cup of boiling water over one teaspoon of cornmeal. Let the mixture sit for five minutes, then add some salt (to personal taste) and drink slowly.

Chapter VIII

Teeth and gums:

Tooth decay and gum disease are common factors leading to offensive breath, premature loss of natural teeth, and general deterioration of overall health resulting from discomfort in masticating foods required to maintain a healthy body. Food residue packed between teeth and under loose gums is a major source of bad breath and can also lead to tooth decay.

The most common cause of tooth decay is consumption of refined sugars used in making sweet desserts and candies. Another major cause is lack of routine oral hygiene including flossing, brushing, tongue scraping, and gargling with an antiseptic mouthwash.

Raw, cold-pressed sesame oil is loaded with vitamin E, calcium, essential fatty acids and other minerals that promote healthy gums and aid in healing of diseased gums. Rinse mouth vigorously with a teaspoon of the oil each morning and before going to bed.

Bleeding, swelling and irritation of gums can be reduced by a vitamin E rinse instead of sesame oil. The liquid can also be massaged into gums with the fingertips for quick relief.

Tea made from peach pits generally does not irritate the gums and will help keep a minor mouth infection from spreading. The tea is mild enough when used as a rinse to clean mouth several times a day until infection clears up.

Three echinacea capsules and one teaspoon of goldenseal tincture taken twice a day beginning as soon as symptoms begin can destroy bacteria causing teeth and gum disease while also strengthening the immune system to better resist harmful bacteria.

The antiseptic properties contained in tea tree oil can help fight infection causing red inflamed gums and toothache. Rub the oil twice daily directly on the sore area in mouth.

Grapefruit seed extract has antibacterial properties which can kill microorganisms damaging teeth and gums. Swab a few drops directly on the affected area three time daily using a cotton swab. Continue treatment until infection vanishes.

For a toothache having more shooting pain

than throbbing pain, drinking Coffea Cruda may provide relief. The coffee is made from unroasted coffee berries and is also reported to provide relief from headache pain.

At the first indication of pain, rub some salt directly on the sensitive area. Salt should kill the bacteria initiating the infection. But, if infection persists, it is best to consult a dentist.

For a mild pain around teeth or gums, chew some whole fresh cloves available from a herb shop or gourmet food store. Chew the cloves on the opposite side of mouth from where the pain is manifested.

When waiting for dental treatment for a toothache, apply moistened comfrey tea bags directly on the affected tooth and adjacent gums. The moist comfrey should reduce pain and swelling making the waiting time more tolerable.

For a cheap and effective mouthwash, rinse mouth thoroughly with a quarter teaspoon of salt mixed into four ounces of water to kill harmful bacteria.

A teaspoon of salt mixed with a teaspoon of baking soda makes an excellent substitute for expensive toothpaste.

To reduce the yellowness of teeth, rub half a ripe strawberry over entire surface of teeth three time a day.

For extra whiteness, frequently rub teeth with a mixture of honey and charcoal.

To whiten stained teeth, mix one cup of strong camomile tea with the fresh juice of one lemon and a quarter cup of white vinegar. Mix a few drops of the resulting liquid into a tablespoon of baking soda and brush teeth at least twice a day.

Rubbing teeth every morning with a clean lemon peel will whiten teeth noticeably.

For overall mouth health, sip frequently on a tea made of chamomile flowers .

Use a sassafras twig for a natural toothbrush. Chew the end of a fresh twig until it is well shredded and use to massage teeth and remove food particles trapped between teeth. The process will leave mouth smelling nice and fresh.

Visual health:

To many, vision is the most devastating sense to lose at any age and there are many eye diseases which can cause pain, discomfort, vision loss and blindness. Some of the best known and most feared eye disorders are cataracts, macular degeneration, glaucoma, and retinal deterioration (from aging). There are many lesser infections, diseases, and irritations of the eyes that can be prevented and treated with diet adjustments, visual hygiene and using food products as home remedies rather than prescription drugs.

There are also many chemical vapors (mostly harmful gases) that pose a danger to vision including smog and other air pollution from energy, agricultural and transportation industries. Eye irritants and visual impairment due to environmental chemical exposure cannot be addressed by diet or self-healing remedies and must be treated by a specialist in optometry. Proper bodily nutrition and home remedies for other minor eye irritations should be considered.

In addition to lack of sufficient sleep, drinking too much alcohol, being allergic to your eye makeup, and contact lens irritation; bloodshot eyes can be caused by a vitamin B-2 (riboflavin) deficiency which can be addressed by 15 mg of vitamin B-2 daily plus a tablespoon of brewer's yeast.

Vitamin B-2 deficiency can also cause cataracts. Brewer's yeast is the richest source of vitamin B-2 (riboflavin). If taking a vitamin B-2 supplement, also take a vitamin B-complex to avoid high urinary losses of B vitamins. Other foods high in vitamin B-2 include broccoli, beans, wheat germ, salmon, turnip tops and beets.

Another "eye vitamin" is vitamin C which helps prevent poor diet damage to the watery portions of eye cells in the cornea and retina. Take 1,000 mg of vitamin C every day or eat foods that contain vitamin C such as broccoli, sweet potatoes, citrus fruits, and bell peppers. Chamomile eye washes are believed to inhibit cataract formation.

Red, watery, itching eyes can be caused by allergies, dust and polluted air; but when the irritation is severe and persistent, the cause may be conjunctivitis (pinkeye) which is quite contagious. One home remedy for pinkeye is to make a fresh poultice of grated apple or grated raw red potato and place on closed eye and let the poultice remain in place for a half hour. Repeat this remedy for two to three days. If condition does not clear up completely, see an eye specialist for professional health care.

Eyebright, (a plant) can also be used to treat pinkeye. Mix three drops of eyebright tincture (available at health food stores) to one tablespoon of just boiled water. When cooled to room temperature, bathe the eye with the mixture. If both eyes are infected, make a fresh mixture for each eye. Conjunctivitis is a highly contagious viral, fungal or allergic infection. Do not continue home remedies more than three days at most before seeing an ophtalmologist (eye doctor).

Goat milk yoghurt may also be used as a poultice for pinkeye. Make a poultice by gently squeezing out excess fluid and place over infected eye(s) for a half hour each day for two to three days. In addition, eat a portion or two of goat milk yoghurt each day. The active culture in the yoghurt provides healthy bacteria in the gastrointestinal tract which fights infections.

Omega-3 fatty acids found in cold water fish and flax seed oil can help relieve dry eyes from tear ducts that do not produce enough fluid. Omega-3 fatty acids increase the viscosity of oils made by the body for the skin and eyes. Correction of the dry eyes problem is more desirable than resorting to artificial tears (eye drops).

For eye inflammation, slice a peeled overripe apple and place the pulp over closed eyes. Secure the poultice in place with a bandage or strip of cloth and let the poultice work for at least a half hour. The poultice can also be made from grated raw potato, freshly mashed papaya pulp, or mashed cooked beets.

For puffy eyes, place used, cool and moist tea bags over closed eyes for a fifteen minute poultice treatment. Repeat each morning as necessary. Another remedy is to crush a tablespoon of fennel seeds and mix into a pint of just boiled water. Let steep and cool for at least fifteen minutes. When liquid cools to room temperature, dip cotton pads into liquid and place over closed

121

eyelids for fifteen minutes.

Another option for eye inflammation is the herb horsetail sold by health food stores. Steep one teaspoon of dried horsetail in hot water for ten minutes. Let cool and dunk cotton pads into liquid and apply to closed eyes for ten minutes. Then redunk the pads and apply for another ten minutes. Wait a half hour and then repeat the process at which time the inflammation should begin to clear up.

For "tired eyes," place freshly sliced cucumbers over closed eyelids for about fifteen minutes to obtain soothing and healing relief. Another remedy is a rosemary tea bag or a teaspoon of loose rosemary in a cup of just-boiled water. Saturate a cotton pad with the mixture and place on closed eyes for fifteen minutes.

The Chemistry of Health   Don Alexander

Sunflower seeds contain vitamins, iron, and calcium believed to be very beneficial for eyes. Eat blueberries in season to help night vision. Eat lots of watercress in salads or drink watercress tea along with carrots (fresh or cooked) to treat night blindness. A handful of shelled sunflower seeds every day helps skiers cope with sun blindness triggered by looking at large expanses of snow or ice for extended periods of time.

To treat sties (a painful red bump on eyelid), place a handful of fresh parsley in a soup bowl. Pour a cup of boiling water overt the parsley and let steep for fifteen minutes. Let cool enough to soak a washcloth in the hot parsley water, lie down, and cover both closed eyes for twenty minutes. Repeat the remedy after a few hours. This treatment also works well for eye puffiness.

A sty results from infection of the oil

glands that service the eyes. Dabbing the sty with castor oil throughout the day will help eliminate the sty.

Chapter IX

Miscellaneous home remedies:

Anemia:

The life of the body is in the blood. Every body cell requires oxygen for normal functioning and replication. Cancer breeds when cellular respiration feeds on sugars rather than oxygen. Red blood cells carry oxygen throughout the body in the form of hemoglobin. When body iron is below normal hemoglobin cannot carry enough oxygen to permit the healthy respiration of oxygen within the trillions of body cells. The result is called anemia and the main symptom is chronic fatigue. Extreme anemia is usually treated by taking iron supplements or by iron infusions if oral ingestion of iron cannot be tolerated.

Anemia can be treated by an iron rich diet containing beef, spinach, unsweetened pure grape juice, watercress, radishes, garlic, kohlrabi, chives, leeks and onions. Snack on dried apricots and raisins. Two tablespoons of raw (not canned) sauerkraut after meals is a highly recommended blood fortifier and highly nutritious. Raw sauerkraut is sold in health food stores.

Arthritis:

Arthritis, rheumatism, bursitis and gout are terms used to describe inflammation or pain in joints, muscles, and fibrous tissues caused primarily by an excess of uric acid in the bloodstream. These ailments which may manifest themselves in over 100 different forms plague approximately 66 million Americans.

Certain vegetables called "nightshade foods" increase the pain and discomfort of many arthritis sufferers. These vegetables are generally classified as white potatoes, eggplants, green peppers and tomatoes. The reason for sensitivity to these nightshade foods has not been definitely established.

Foods that are reported by arthritis sufferers to ease arthritic conditions are healthy portions of cherries, cherry juice, fresh string beans (whole or juiced), half cup of parsley juice before each meal, celery, gin-soaked raisins, apple cider vinegar mixed with equal parts of honey, two glasses of grape juice daily, corn silk tea, juice of a large lime squeezed into a cup of black coffee, and herbal teas made with sage, rosemary, nettles, and basil. These foods and herbs act as pain relief and dilute the uric acid in the blood.

Atherosclerosis:

Atherosclerosis is a mind numbing term for clogging of the arteries caused by deposits of fatty substances, cholesterol, calcium and other forms of plaque over time connected with poor diet, lack of physical exercise and smoking. Professional health care should be sought for advanced atherosclerosis, but there are also dietary recommendations that will reduce cholesterol levels and help reduce the risks of stroke and heart attack.

Garlic is reported to help clear arteries by removing toxic waste. Two garlic cloves minced into a half glass of orange juice and swallowed without chewing will avoid "garlic breath." This should be a daily routine to both cleanse arteries and lower bad cholesterol level.

Rutin in bioflavonoids is necessary for proper absorption of vitamin C. Taking 500 mg of rutin daily with 500 mg of vitamin C should strengthen capillaries and arterial walls, help prevent hemorrhaging and fight atherosclerosis.

The only foods containing cholesterol are animal products (meat, poultry, fish and dairy products). Reducing or eliminating these cholesterol loaded foods from the diet is a perfect way to lower bad cholesterol as well as avoid a host of related health issues connected with these particular food items.

Eat half an avocado every day to lower cholesterol by as much as 42%. The fat in avocados is monounsaturated which is beneficial and the tasty tropical fruit also contains thirteen essential minerals including iron, copper, potassium and magnesium.

Two large apples a day can drop cholesterol by up to 16%. Apples are rich in flavonoids and pectin which may form a gel in the stomach which keeps fats from being totally absorbed.

Two raw carrots a day have been reported to reduce cholesterol by approximately 11%.

Kiwi fruit for an energy boosting, cholesterol lowering afternoon snack also delivers magnesium, potassium and fiber.

Omega-3 fatty acids break down cholesterol in the lining of blood vessels and are contained in abundance in cold water fish (such as salmon and mackerel), and flax seed oil.

Hoarseness/laryngitis:

Drink a mixture of two teaspoons of onion juice and one teaspoon of honey; or drink a cup of hot peppermint tea with a teaspoon of honey every three hours until condition improves.

Peel and mince a bulb of garlic. Cover the minced garlic with honey and let stand for about two hours. Then, take a teaspoon of the garlic and honey treatment every hour without chewing the garlic to avoid garlic breath.

Grate a handful of radishes and squeeze them through cheese cloth to get the radish juice. Then slowly swallow a teaspoon of the juice every half hour.

For treatment of tonsillitis, see a physician. In the meanwhile, bake one medium banana in its skin at 350 degrees for 30 minutes. Peel the banana and mash while adding one tablespoon of extra-virgin cold-pressed olive oil. Spread the mush on a clean strip of cloth and wrap the cloth around the neck at shoulders. Leave wrap around neck 30 minutes morning and evening.

Constipation:

Natural remedies are preferred over commercial chemical laxatives which can kill beneficial bacteria, retard the absorption of vital nutrients, stuff up intestinal walls, and get rid of necessary vitamins and minerals. These commercial laxatives can also become habit forming when used too frequently, and can actually cause constipation rather than relieve the condition. Chronic constipation should be analyzed by a physician. For occasional constipation, there are some favorite home remedies:

Before breakfast, drink the juice of half a

lemon in a cup of warm water sweetened with honey.

Eat or drink one of the food items below at room temperature:

six ounces of prune juice, five stewed prunes, papaya, two peeled apples, six to eight dried figs soaked overnight in glass of water (in morning, drink water, eat figs).

Two hours after evening meal, eat an apple, a peach and an apricot.

Scrub two raw beets and eat raw in the morning. This should produce a bowel movement in about twelve hours.

Flax seed is reported to promote regularity. Eat two tablespoons and drink a quart of water. Sunflower seeds are also recommended for constipation. Eat a half cup of shelled raw and unsalted seeds and drink a quart of water.

Drink a warm 8 ounce glass of sauerkraut juice followed immediately by an 8 ounce glass of unsweetened grapefruit juice. Then, stay close to the necessary room.

One teaspoon of wheat germ and one teaspoon of brewer's yeast with each meal should trigger a bowel movement.

Not only is olive oil good for lowering cholesterol but taking a teaspoon of extra-virgin, cold-pressed olive oil in the morning and one hour after eating should relieve constipation.

Eat persimmons (in season) to promote regularity.

Add raw unprocessed bran to your morning

cereal. Start with one teaspoon of bran and increase gradually each morning up to two tablespoons (stop increasing the bran when you find the bran/cereal mix that works for you).

Eat raw escarole or boil in water and drink the water.   Roast Spanish onion and eat at bedtime.

Eat garlic every day or take odorless garlic supplement.

Raw spinach contains lots of vitamins and minerals and is also a mild natural laxative. Wash raw spinach thoroughly before eating to avoid food-borne parasites.

For a stool softener, soak a tablespoon of raisins or three prunes in water for two hours and then eat the raisins or prunes before eating evening meal.

Diabetes:

Diabetes results from the failure of the pancreas to produce enough insulin to burn up the body's intake of sugars and starches from foods eaten. Common symptoms of diabetes are frequent urination and constant thirst. Other symptoms are feeling weak, tired and lightheaded. Individuals experiencing such symptoms should see a physician to be checked for diabetes and appropriate treatment.

In addition to professional health care, there are some home remedies that can help cope with diabetes:

Generally speaking, a low calorie, high-carbohydrate diet combined with a brisk half hour walk after each meal is highly recommended by physicians treating diabetes.

Blood sugar for some diabetics can be lowered by one to two tablespoons of organic, extra-virgin coconut oil. A daily helping of watercress, garlic and parsley can also help regulate blood sugar levels for some diabetics.

Diarrhea:

Diarrhea can be caused by several factors including overeating, a bacterial, viral or parasitic infection, mild food poisoning, personal anxiety and excessive fatigue. Diarrhea depletes the body of potassium, magnesium, and perhaps sodium which often results in fatigue, depression and dehydration. When suffering from diarrhea, increase the intake of clear fluids. Chronic diarrhea is indicative of a serious health problem and bloody diarrhea should be immediately evaluated by a physician.

Some self-help remedies reported to be effective are:

A pinch of allspice mixed in a cup of warm water; or a double pinch of cinnamon plus a pinch of powdered cloves in a warm cup of milk; or two cups of boiled water with a pinch of cayenne pepper and quarter teaspoon of cinnamon (after cooling, drink a quarter cup of mixture every thirty minutes until the two cups are consumed.

Prepare two tablespoons of onion juice and take each hour with a cup of peppermint tea to relieve diarrhea. Eating cooked rice flavored with cinnamon may also help ease diarrhea.

Ear wax buildup:

Prepare one tablespoon of warm corn oil and sprinkle the oil with black pepper. Dip a cotton wad into the peppered oil and carefully insert the cotton into the ear. Remove the cotton after ten minutes and repeat the treatment for the other ear.

Squeeze ten drops of warm 3% hydrogen peroxide into ear and let the the hydrogen peroxide work for a five minutes. Tilt head and drain ear into a tissue. Then, carefully remove softened wax with cotton wad. Repeat treatment for the other ear.

Prepare two teaspoons of warm sesame oil, tilt head and put one teaspoon in right ear using eyedropper, then plug ear with cotton ball. Put the other teaspoon full into the left ear and plug likewise. Let oil soften wax for ten minutes, then flush ears with warm water using a squeeze bulb.

Ringing in the ears:

Continuous ringing in the ears (tinnitus) is a very difficult problem to diagnose. The precise cause is unknown. Some causes are believed to be noise-induced hearing loss, ear infection, cardiovascular disease, jaw misalignment, wax buildup, and an overdose of salicylate contained in some drugs including aspirin. Instead of constant ringing, some individuals suffering with tinnitus may hear clicking, roaring, whistling, or hissing. Drug induced tinnitus should stop when the offending drug is discontinued. Some home remedies recommended by those suffering with tinnitus are:

Use a heating pad on both hands and feet to redistribute blood circulation which reduces pressure in congested areas (perhaps in the ears).

With eyedropper, squeeze four drops of castor oil in each ear and plug ears with cotton balls. Leave ears plugged overnight. Remove cotton in the morning and drain oil from ears, then flush with warm water squirted through a squeeze bulb.

Prepare six peeled garlic cloves (large), and one cup of almond oil. Blend the garlic with the oil until cloves are minced into tiny pieces. Clean a glass jar with boiling water and dry the jar. Pour garlic and oil mixture into the jar and cover jar. Put jar in refrigerator for seven days, then strain the liquid from jar into an eyedropper bottle. Each night, warm a small amount of the liquid and put three drops in each ear and plug ears with cotton balls. Remove cotton and flush ears in the morning. Keep the liquid refrigerated and do not use same liquid after one month.

Hearing loss:

Hearing loss is reported to be helped dramatically by stewing a mixture of garlic cloves and olive oil, then straining and pressing out the liquid and putting four drops in each ear and plugging with cotton overnight. Repeat this treatment on a daily basis for at least seven days.

Brisk walking or bicycling can help age-related hearing loss and hearing loss from loud noises. The exercise is reported by researchers to improve hearing by circulating blood to inner ear cells thus supplying the cells with more oxygen and increasing the supply of chemicals that protect the cells.

Drinking one ounce of garlic juice mixed with one ounce of onion juice daily is reported to improve hearing. Be prepared to get some strange looks from people close enough to smell your breath. A glass of tomato juice after one hour may help the odor.

Headaches:

Headaches may be a warning that something is wrong with bodily functions which needs to be diagnosed by a physician. Headaches can also be caused by fatigue, anxiety, depression, nervous tension, constipation, lack of sleep, dread of some pending event or action that needs to be taken, and side effects of various medications. For persistent headaches it is highly advisable to see a physician. For occasional headaches from identified causes, there are some self-help remedies that do not have the side effects associated with various over-the-counter and prescribed medications:

Eat a couple dozen almonds instead of taking medication. Almonds contain salicylates which is the pain relieving ingredient in aspirin. Almonds are exceptionally good for your body anyway and two dozen almonds contain around 200 calories making an almond snack a moderate calorie treat.

Rub some essence of rosemary oil on forehead, temples and behind ears and then inhale the fumes from the bottle several times. If headache doesn't fade in a half hour, repeat the rubbing and inhaling.

Combine one teaspoon of dried basil with one cup of water. Bring to boil, remove from stove and add two tablespoons of witch hazel. Cool the mixture and then dunk a washcloth in it. Wring out the cloth and apply to forehead with bandage. Keep bandage in place until headache subsides.

Grate a red potato or apple and make a poultice. Bandage to forehead and let poultice work for two hours.

The Chemistry of Health   Don Alexander

Mix half a teaspoon of angelica with three quarters cup of hot water and drink. The pain should be diminished and you may feel delightful.

While dressed warmly except for bare feet, stroll back and forth in an ankle deep tub of really cold water. When feet began to feel warm, step out of tub, dry feet and go straight to bed. Cover up and relax until headache disappears.

Boil one cup of apple cider vinegar mixed in one cup of water. When fumes begin to rise, remove pot from stove, cover head with a towel, bend over pot, then inhale and exhale through nose deeply while counting slowly to one hundred.

Eat a bowl of fresh strawberries. They contain salicylates, a natural pain killer. Lie down in a dark, quiet room.

Hemorrhoids:

Hemorrhoids afflict, at one time or another, 67% of Americans and can be a definite pain in the rectum. For those prone to suffer hemorrhoids, it is recommended to avoid foods containing white flour and refined sugar. Alcohol should also be eliminated from routine ingestion. Drink lots of fruit and vegetable juices plus load up on fruits and vegetables every meal. Take a half hour walk twice daily and do not strain or hold breath while having a bowel movement. Other favorite self-help remedies include:

Eat four raw unprocessed almonds every day and chew each almond to a fine mush.

Apply liquid lecithin directly on hemorrhoids each day until they heal up.

Make a poultice of finely chopped cranberries and place over hemorrhoids and keep in place with padded shorts or panties. Leave in place for a couple of hours to relieve pain and help heal inflamed hemorrhoids.

Boil a large leek for a daily snack between meals or with evening meal.

Carve an ice cube into suppository shape and insert into anus. This should reduce swelling and help heal hemorrhoids.

Saturate a clean cotton wad with papaya juice and bandage in place over hemorrhoids. Leave in place between bowel movements. This should reduce bleeding and irritation of anus.

To help prevent the incidence of hemorrhoids, increase the fiber and fluid content of daily diet and eat four raw almonds every day plus a brisk half hour walk.

Leg cramps:

Leg cramps are often caused by a deficiency in various nutritional essentials such as protein, calcium, magnesium, vitamin E, or potassium. To reduce the frequency of leg cramps, eat plenty of leafy green vegetables and avoid fatty meats, sugar and white flour.

Using a chemical diuretic rather than a natural substitute may cause an excessive loss of potassium thereby causing leg cramps. Try eating a banana twice daily and switch to healthy foods that have diuretic properties such as cucumbers, lettuce and celery and try to get off chemical diuretic.

Quinine is prescribed to relieve leg cramps. Drinking a glass of tonic water (which contains quinine) may help calm leg cramps.

Cramp bark is a herb that earns its name

and is available at health food stores. Take two teaspoons every three hours as needed.

Nightly leg cramps may be relieved by one tablespoon of calcium lactate mixed with one teaspoon of apple cider vinegar and one teaspoon of honey stirred in a half glass of warm water.

One cup of red raspberry-leaf tea both morning and evening ingested daily can ward off leg cramps.

A daily vitamin B-6 supplement may help with leg cramps. Vitamin E taken before each meal may also help. Check with physician for dosage recommendation. Drinking at least 8 ounces of water before bedding down for the night may also add to leg cramp relief.

Warts:

Warts are generally believed to be caused by some type of virus and appear primarily on hands, face and feet but can actually appear anywhere (just ask Bill Clinton) including inside nose. Some at home, self-help remedies that come highly recommended are:

Apply used tea bag to wart for fifteen minutes daily.

Rub the inside skin of a pineapple on wart morning and evening until wart disappears.

Grate a carrot and mix with teaspoon of olive oil and apply to wart twice daily for half an hour.

Break the stems on some dandelions and squeeze out a little juice, then apply to wart morning and evening for one week.

Mash a fresh fig until mushy and apply to wart half an hour each day until wart is gone.

Bandage a fresh slice of raw potato or garlic clove on wart and leave in place over night and repeat daily for one week. If wart does not disappear, try another of the above remedies.

The Chemistry of Health   Don Alexander